DMT Machine Elves

A Journey Into The World Of The Dmt Spirit
With Fascinating Theories About Entities.

i

Title:
DMT Machine Elves

Subtitle
A Journey Into The World Of The Dmt Spirit With Fascinating Theories About Entities.

TABLE OF CONTENT

INTRODUCTION

Dimethyltryptamine, also known as DMT, is one of the most potent hallucinogenic chemicals that can be found on Earth.

Our view of time and space can be warped by this combination, yet it can also extend the mind in ways that you would never have imagined were conceivable.

The encounter of "beings" that appear to reside within the domain of DMT is one of the many peculiarly prevalent experiences that people have when they are under the influence of DMT.

The term "machine elves" or "DMT entities" is more generally used to refer to these types of beings. They give off the impression of being conscious, independent, and just as curious about us as we are about them.

There is a lot of controversy over the existence of these mystery entities. The DMT is a tool that enables us to view and interact with things that exist in another dimension, according to some people, while others believe that these effects are only fictitious side effects of the drug.

This book will discuss different hypotheses concerning the origins of DMT machine elves, covering both the mystical and scientific causes for their existence.

What Are DMT Elves?

People who live in psychedelic hyperspace are known as DMT elves. These elves are essentially humanoid creatures. Only when people take extremely high doses of DMT, known as breakthrough doses, do they experience them.

Concerning their origins, there are a lot of concerns that need to be answered; are they people that live in another dimension? Are they the souls or spirits of people who have lived in the past? Angels or divine beings are they, respectively? Another possibility is that they are the result of our innate propensity to recognize human motifs in patterns that are otherwise devoid of significance.

There have been some intriguing attempts to classify these beings to have a better understanding of what they are, but nobody understands where they come from.

Terence McKenna, who passed away recently, was one of the most influential psychedelic explorers, writers, philosophers, and ethnobotanists who ever lived. He was also the one who came up with the term "DMT elves."

McKenna, along with a large number of other psychonauts, has reported that they were "greeted" by some unknown creatures when they were on a breakthrough DMT trip.

It would appear that these beings are sentient and independent. They will talk with you, observe you, show you various objects or locations, and will occasionally even pull small pranks on you or taunt you. They will try to communicate with you.

In his book Archaic Revival, McKenna was the first person to refer to these species as "self-transforming machine elves." His observations revealed that they were not dissimilar to the classic elves or leprechauns that are seen in legend. Beings that are continuously changing their forms and transforming their appearance are little, lively, and almost childlike.

During the 1970s, Terence McKenna and his brother Dennis McKenna embarked on a journey to the Amazon to gain an understanding of the regional utilization of psychedelic plants. Terence was taken aback when he discovered that local shamans had images that were comparable to his own. It was said that the shamans had a meeting with a small group of people who would provide them with valuable information that they could bring back to the real world.

Different Names For DMT Machine Elves

- Divine Beings

- Fractal Elves

- Angels or Spirits

- DMT Entities

- Self-Transforming Machine Elves

- Clockwork Elves

- DMT Aliens

- Tykes

Some peculiar commonalities coincide with a number of these tales, even though the descriptions of DMT elves might differ from one individual to the next.

In addition to being portrayed as kind, playful, and prankish, these beings are sometimes described as being annoying. Despite possessing intelligence that is beyond the comprehension of our human minds, they have the innocence of a child. They can teleport themselves and the psychedelic guests to new regions, as well as the ability to morph and change shape at will. In one sense, they are all-powerful. They can communicate complicated concepts to us.

The fact that the majority of persons who come into contact with these creatures are in agreement that they have some kind of goal (although it is not clear what that purpose might be) is one of the most intriguing aspects of these beings.

It is virtually always the case that the machine elves have something significant to demonstrate to us, but how individuals perceive their acts might differ substantially. They may criticize or make fun of us for features of our personalities that we are not proud of. Sometimes they appear to be malevolent. On the other hand, in the end, this criticism is seen as a constructive catalyst for changing unfavorable characteristics of one's nature.

Sometimes machine elves are humorous and offer positive insights into challenges that we encounter in our own lives or society. Other times, they are serious problem solvers.

DMT ENTITIES & ONTOLOGICAL SHOCK

One thing is certain, even though it is not obvious whether these beings are genuine or not: when we come into contact with a DMT entity, even if it is only once, our perspective on life and death can be altered irrevocably.

A condition of ontological shock is frequently experienced when one comes into contact with intelligent and sentient beings that appear to be from another dimension and are in some way able to impart knowledge regarding life, death, and the nature of reality.

It is possible to have an ontological shock when one is compelled to reevaluate their entire viewpoint on something.

The results of a survey that was administered to 2561 individuals who had either smoked or vaporized DMT were evaluated in a study that was published in the Journal of Psychopharmacology in the year 2020. While approximately twenty-five percent of the people who participated in this study stated that they were atheists before the encounter, only ten percent of the people who participated in the survey believed themselves to be atheists at the time of the survey.

Rick Strassman, who was the first person to research DMT that was permitted by the Drug Enforcement Administration (DEA) in the 1990s, was baffled by the number of contacts that his subjects had with entities that were associated with DMT.

Listed below are some of the other fascinating discoveries that were made by this research:

1. One hundred and ninety-nine percent of those who come into contact with DMT entities display a powerful emotional reaction during the encounter.

2. A significant proportion of individuals had a favorable perception of the creatures, with 96 percent identifying them as intelligent, 96 percent as benign, 78 percent as sacred, and

34 percent as helpful. Only 11 percent of individuals categorized the beings as "malicious."

3. When individuals encounter DMT entities, around 66 percent of them are provided either a message or a task.

4. The interaction was described as feeling "more real than reality" by 81% of those who participated in the survey.

5. The majority of responders (almost 90 percent) believe that the experience resulted in long-term enhancements to their well-being and overall pleasure with life.

What Do DMT Entities Look Like?

Because of the speed and intensity with which they transform into other forms, it is famously difficult to define the physical look of machine elves.

In addition to this, they are frequently composed entirely of fractal shapes and intricate geometric patterns, both of which are in a state of perpetual change and in the process of developing into new patterns.

A number of individuals perceive these things as animal forms, while others perceive them as traditional aliens in the spirit of science fiction.

14

These entities are said to be humanoid, sentient, and to reside in a universe where everything is composed of fractal patterns, according to the consensus which has been reached.

What Do DMT Elves Do?

Even though the visualizations that are a result of DMT are notable, it is the spiritual elements of the trip that are possibly the most significant, and Strassman is the only one who can express this influence better than he does. He states that "the role of the creatures is to communicate," and that the information that they transmit is what they communicate. Their shape or form may contain that information; but, what is more significant is that there is an interaction between the observer and the creatures, which can be vocal or nonverbal at times. After that, it is up to our minds and our intellects to understand the message and to derive meaning from it.

Strassman's perspective is reinforced by data that was compiled from studies that were conducted recently, such as the Davis research. The majority of people who use DMT engage with its spirits through emotional, intuitive, and telepathic ways, according to the research conducted by Davis. These mechanical elves frequently have a sense of realism, as if they were the judges of a profound and concealed reality. Many people claim that having them is a defining moment or a life-altering event, with a significant influence on their state of mind, their overall wellness, and their perspective on life.

ARE DMT ALIENS REAL?

Not only is there no evidence that DMT entities are genuine, but there is also no evidence that they are not real. Without a doubt, we will never know.

The question that arises here is, "What exactly does it mean to be real?"

Ontology is the name of the subfield of metaphysics that is directly concerned with this subject. One can determine what is deemed real and what is considered imaginary by determining the ontological status of anything.

The following are two schools of thought concerning what is real and what is imaginary that could be utilized to establish whether or not DMT creatures are real or the result of imagination:

1. Physicalism (DMT Elves Aren't Real)

When it comes to reality, everything that has a physical form is real, whereas everything else is fictional. It is necessary for anything to entail visible phenomena for it to exist.

To put it another way, we need to be able to determine whether or not something exists by utilizing either our own eyes or scientific devices such as a telescope or a microscope. Therefore, anything that cannot be viewed or detected in the physical world is considered to be imaginary (not real).

According to this concept, entities that consist of DMT are not real since they do not have a physical form that can be observed.

2. Idealism (DMT Elves Are Real)

The mind of the observer is the sole source of that which constitutes reality.

According to this criterion, DMT entities are considered to be real if they are experienced. For them to exist, a physical manifestation is not required.

At the moment when you are experiencing something, it is the most genuine it can be. According to all reports, whatever sensation you are having is a genuine one. When you are there, you are experiencing it right now. There is no reason to believe that something did not take place simply because it is no longer present after you return from the vacation.

When you are in a dream, everything that is happening to you is happening. This is also true for dreams. At this very now, you are participating in experiences that are taking place in the present moment. It is not until you awaken that you become aware that what you have been experiencing was a dream, which is distinct from the reality that we encounter when we are awake.

There are a lot of people who say that the experience of taking DMT is "more real than reality itself." It is almost as if the reality that we encounter daily is a delusion, and the realm of DMT is the actual reality.

QUALITIES OF THE DMT DIMENSION

The DMT realm also referred to as "psychedelic hyperspace," is home to beings that are associated with DMT.

If you have never tried DMT previously, there is a particular aspect of this location that you must comprehend.

Without a doubt, the location that DMT transports you to (regardless of where that may be) is both geometric and chaotic. Infinite fractals and patterns that are always shifting make up its composition.

The further you delve into the subject, the more intricate the geometry becomes.

Within the context of his presentation on the hyperbolic geometry of the DMT experience, Andrés Gómez Emilsson, who is affiliated with the Qualia Research Institute, provides an outstanding explanation of this.

Using the geometry of the experience, Emilsson and his colleagues are working on developing a system that will allow them to measure the level of depth that the DMT experience provides. The researchers believe that they will be able to determine the extent of the experience in the DMT world if they can determine the amount of complexity of the geometric patterns that they encounter while on the DMT trip.

Six separate layers of the DMT realm are listed by the Qualia Research Institute, which are as follows:

1. At the threshold, the initial effects of DMT include improved high-definition vision and colors that are more vivid.
2. Chrysanthemum is the emergence of a textured fabric that is composed of complex symmetrical forms and vibrant colors (often looks like a chrysanthemum flower).
3. The chrysanthemum is the source of the Magic Eye, which develops into a sophisticated autostereogram over time.
4. The waiting room is a room that is created by the autostereogram that surrounds you and creates a space for you to sit and wait for a bit before going on to the next step.

5. The curvature of the geometric patterns changes to such an extreme degree that topological bifurcations occur uncontrollably. This is known as a breakthrough.

6. Amnesia is a level of amnesia that is so severe that it causes you to completely have no awareness of your physical existence.

At the breakthrough stage, DMT entities are often met for the first time.

What Causes DMT Hallucinations?

What exactly is the reason behind the prevalence of these "entities" in DMT experiences remains a mystery. However, Strassman can give insight after conducting a study for several decades. "The only things that people can envision are those that they have previously seen or experienced," he explains. The component pieces can rearrange themselves in a variety of different ways; but, it is necessary for those parts to already exist in the subject's mind. Various hues, forms, and motion. We can sense things that are typically invisible, and those things need to be made present in an apparent form, that we can identify, regardless of how weird they may be.

Psychedelics, especially DMT, help us perceive these things.

This new generation of neuroscience research is progressively uncovering surprising layers of how humans experience consciousness; the study of DMT and other psychedelic substances may prove to be a vital aspect of this larger research. Strassman's work is a complement to this new wave of research. On the other hand, in contrast to psilocybin and LSD, the human body naturally manufactures its own DMT. Furthermore, according to several speculative medical ideas, this endogenous DMT could be involved in the process of constructing the world that we experience when we are awake every day.

SOME THEORIES ABOUT DMT ENTITIES

One cannot tell for certain whether or if DMT beings exist, where they originate, or even what they desire from humans. There is no way to know for certain.

The following are eight hypotheses that are currently being discussed on the possible nature of these creatures and the origins of their existence.

Regard all of this with a healthy dose of skepticism. All of them are only hypotheses or concepts that are enjoyable to contemplate; but, there is no way to confirm or deny any of them, regardless of how absurd they may appear to be.

Theory One: Denizens of the DMT Realm

According to Terence McKenna's conceptualization of machine elves, this appears to be the idea that most closely matches his understanding.

The psychedelic sphere of consciousness is said to be inhabited by the DMT creatures that human beings come into contact with.

In addition, you might make a connection between this and the concept of a "spirit realm," which is a place where various types of sentient consciousness dwell but are unable to interact with the physical world as we know it. To enter this world, one must either be in a deep state of meditation or be under the influence of hallucinogenic substances (which have a surprising amount of overlap with the psychedelic experience).

There are many similarities between the conventional notion of elves, fairies, and leprechauns from legend and the DMT elves that are found in the world. Small and mischievous, they possess a variety of magical skills, including the ability to change their appearance, teleport, and communicate with others.

There are a wide variety of personalities and subcategories, just like there are millions of people. Some are benign, innocent, and kind, whereas others are hostile and selfish.

There is a possibility that there is a civilization of creatures that reside in another world that can only be accessed by altering the frequency of awareness. The use of DMT and other psychedelic substances allows us to occasionally visit their domain, whereas the only way for them to enter ours is through a shift in awareness that is analogous to what we experience.

Theory Two: The Human Brain as a Consciousness Generator

Many of the hypotheses that are provided in this article are mystical explanations for the entities that are associated with DMT; however, there is also a scientific explanation.

One may make the case that the brain is nothing more than a conduit for the production of awareness. Specifically, it is responsible for converting the sensory information that we get from the environment around us into experience.

Existence is already intrinsically disordered and unpredictable. For us to be able to interact with it, we need to find a means to eliminate the background noise.

To do this, the default mode network (DMN) is comprised of several brain areas that are linked to one another and collaborate. In addition to regulating the communication between different brain systems, it is in charge of filtering the information that is taken in by the brain.

It is via the DMN that we can establish a connection with the world around us by defining fundamental features of existence, such as the distinction between "self" and "other." The default mode network (DMN) is frequently referred to as the physical location of the "ego," which is vital to our survival since it serves as the anchoring point.

The 5HT2A receptor is activated by DMT and other psychedelic substances, which is how they produce their psychedelic effects. Because of this receptor, the effects of the DMN are muted, which leads to an influx of information within the brain that would typically be filtered out.

The so-called "DMT hyperspace" and the creatures that are contained inside it might very well be formed totally from our brains. This is a possibility that cannot be discounted. Because DMT alters the characteristics of the consciousness generator that is the human brain, we can experience what appears to be another realm. However, we are experiencing the same information that is being translated differently within the brain.

Take into consideration a computer monitor. The purpose of this device is to retrieve data from a computer and transform it into the visual representation that we see on the screen. Changing just a few lines of code allows the monitor to take identical information and utilize it to display a wide variety of twisted and discolored forms and projections instead of the original information. It is only how the monitor interprets the data, and this does not imply that these forecasts are true.

Theory Three: Alien Communication

According to this hypothesis, the creatures and experiences that we have while under the influence of DMT are messages that have been sent to us by some kind of extraterrestrial species. The information included in these signals may include new ideas or insights into emerging technologies, which may subsequently be taken back and distributed to the rest of civilization. Sometimes, it is more of a personal nature.

The appearance of life on other planets is completely unknown to us.

Is it possible that there are beings in the cosmos that are so unlike us that we are unable to even engage in physical contact with them?

Perhaps our human brains just aren't capable of comprehending them due to their complexity.

A good illustration of this would be the fact that our three-dimensional selves would be unable to even comprehend these extraterrestrial beings if they were from the fourth dimension.

In the same way that a being that is just two-dimensional would be unable to even conceive of what the three-dimensional plane might be, three-dimensional creatures are unable to fathom what the plane that is four-dimensional looks like.

The psychedelic experience is the medium via which the DMT alien communication theory proposes that extraterrestrial creatures might interact with humans (as well as dreams). In this area, they can communicate information in the form of visual language, which is a notion that is essential to the experience of being a DMT creature.

Theory Four: The Psychedelic Microscope

Some hypotheses propose that DMT and other psychedelics are similar to a tool that allows us to view something already present, but that we are unable to perceive with our typical human hardware. The notion behind this is the same as that of utilizing a telescope or a microscope.

If you look at a surface that has been well-cleaned, you will not notice any live beings. Nevertheless, if you examine the same surface through the lens of a microscope, you will see that it is teeming with life.

Even though we were unable to see them, those microscopic germs and protozoa were always present as well.

When we use DMT as a kind of microscope, we can view living forms that are constantly present but that we are unable to perceive with our waking human awareness.

An additional comparison that is analogous to that of a radio receiver in the same overall sense.

We can pick up transmissions from radio stations that are running on a certain channel when we have the radio set correctly. We must adjust the frequency of the receiver to be able to make use of the streaming service provided by another radio station.

Is it possible that DMT can alter the frequency of our awareness, so enabling us to tune in to information from other "channels"?

Theory Five: Contact With The Divine

The primary purpose for which psychedelics were utilized was in religious rites and rituals. Ayahuasca, magic mushrooms, salvia, and peyote were some of the substances that were utilized to establish a connection between the shaman and the holy. Even though the meaning of the word "divine" varies from culture to culture, the concept itself remains the same.

Many individuals have the experience of encountering what they perceive to be angels, God, Buddha, Gaia, Krishna, or other beings that are religious or spiritual. At times, people see a deity or spirit that is utterly unconnected to their spiritual ideas, while other times, they see something that is most in line with their spiritual beliefs.

There may be a creator who is all-powerful and who is looking down on us from that heavenly vantage point. They may share a few nuggets of knowledge with us, either to assist society as a whole or for the purpose of assisting in the improvement of the circumstances of a particular individual.

Without the use of psychedelics or DMT, there have been a variety of different sorts of encounters with various forms of the divine. However, these medications appear to have a propensity to induce them more on our terms, which is another thing to consider.

The process is comparable to arranging a meeting with the divine. Although there is no assurance that they will show up, the meeting has been arranged, and the boardroom has been reserved for their presence.

Theory Six: Tapping into the Collective Unconscious

For the first time, Carl Jung put up the concept of the collective unconscious. According to this hypothesis, every single species of human being can reach a realm of awareness that extends beyond our particular experiences.

In some type of ethereal database, the thoughts, experiences, and recollections of individuals who lived before us are preserved. We bring pieces of these experiences with us when we are born at the beginning of our lives.

Certain memories have a practical purpose, such as teaching a newborn infant how to crawl up to its mother's breast for feeding within the first few minutes after birth.

Although certain memories are not necessarily useful, they continue to have an impact on who we are, as well as how we think and behave. These recollections are completely apart from an individual's conscious experience. They are present in our brains, quietly affecting our ideas and behaviors, but they are just out of reach for us to be able to recognize them with conscious awareness. Because of this, Jung referred to it as the collective unconscious on many occasions.

He conceived the idea of shadow labor as a means of revealing one's unconscious pressures and effects. These days, psychedelics are seen as an essential component of this process because they are so powerful in removing concepts and thoughts that are buried deep within the unconscious.

Does the presence of DMT elves represent the manifestation of the collective unconscious?

There is a possibility that this is the reason why machine elves are so eager to offer us the knowledge that has a direct impact on society and why they have so many characteristics with one another.

Theory Seven: Innate Anthropomorphic Recognition

The human species has the intrinsic ability to recognize any humanistic data that may be present in patterns that are otherwise chaotic or random.

Because of this, the inkblot tests that are considered to be conventional for Rorschach most frequently resemble the faces of other people or animals. The occurrence of this phenomenon is documented regardless of the culture from which the observer originates.

Machine elves may be the consequence of the mind having the ability to recognize what looks to be humanoid shapes or faces inside fractal patterns that are otherwise highly random and chaotic.

Theory Eight: Meme Theory

The term "meme" was first used by Richard Dawkins in his book "The Selfish Gene," which was published in 1976. The Greek word mine served as the basis for his creation of the phrase, which he abbreviated to make it more nearly resemble the word "gene."

As defined by the scientific community, a meme is an idea, habit, or talent that is passed down from one person to another through the process of imitation.

The transfer of cultural practices, language, and key technology such as automobiles and clothes are all examples of memes that may be found on a macro scale.

However, likely, the experience of the machine elves is also a meme. Memes are concepts that are transmitted from one person to another (specifically, Terence McKenna), and then they present themselves in the psychedelic experience of other individuals.

It would appear that Rick Doblin is of the opinion that this is the case since he had an interview with Lex Clips in the middle of the year 2021. He thinks that machine elves are a creation of Terence McKenna, which then causes others to experience them once the notion has been passed on.

This does not explain the experiences that have been described by individuals who claim to have had no prior knowledge of the entities linked with DMT before having those experiences.

COMMUNICATING WITH MACHINE ELVES

When individuals come into contact with machine elves, the majority of them report that they acquired some kind of knowledge or insight. However, these entities do not interact with one another using the language that is commonly used. Synesthesia is how they converse with one another. However, rather than hearing it, you see it. They communicate by noise.

This is what Terence McKenna refers to as translinguistic glossolalia, which is another term for communication that is illogical. Because it is so unlike the language and communication that is often used, it is extremely difficult to adequately describe or duplicate.

According to McKenna, this particular sort of visual language is an essential component of the DMT universe. He thought that this visual language was the most comprehensive type of information:

The language that transforms into the thing that it describes and that it is.

It makes it possible to convey information that is extremely complicated without the possibility of it being misunderstood under any circumstances.

DMT Entity Trip Reports

The number of trip reports that describe people having encounters with entities while smoking, vaping, or ingesting DMT is not difficult to locate.

The fact that Joe Rogan claims to have encountered these creatures on one of his DMT trips is something that he discusses on his podcast while having a conversation with Michael Malice.

The following is a selection of DMT trip reports that involve DMT entities. The purpose of this is to offer some background for the variety of ways in which these beings manifest themselves.

- **Trip Report #1: DMT Entities**

(This is one of the trip reports that Terence McKenna has written, in which he meets beings associated with DMT.)

As I fell to the ground, I sank. I [experienced] this hallucination of tumbling forward into these fractal geometric spaces made of light and then I found myself in the equivalent of the Pope's private chapel and insect elf machines were proffering strange little tablets with strange writing on them, and I was aghast, completely appalled, because [in] a matter of seconds... my entire expectation of the nature of the world was just being shredded in front of me. In all honesty, I've never been able to get over it.

It was a colored language that these self-transforming machine elf beings were communicating in. This language condensed into whirling machines that resembled Fabergé eggs but were made out of luminous superconducting ceramics and liquid crystal gels. I mean, it felt like my entire intellectual universe was turning inside out! All of this material was just so strange, so foreign, and so incomprehensible in English that it was a massive surprise.

- **Trip Report #2: DMT Entities**

My field of perception was filled with fractals of a royal purple color. The sensation was similar to that of staring through a kaleidoscope, and the beauty of these sights increased with each passing instant. Not long after that, I was visited by three blue people, two of whom appeared to be male, and one of whom was unquestionably a female. It appeared as though the female was the "leader" of the group; she was standing in front of the other two and was gesturing me in her direction. She was not of this earth, yet she had a human-like form. However, her head was triangular, almost like a spade. One of the angles on her head was in the direction of the north, while the other two angles were due east and west. She intended to demonstrate something to me, and she was beckoning me to come closer.

Unfortunately, in the excitement of using DMT for the first time, none of us thought to turn off the telephone ringer, and the phone rang many times while I was experiencing the effects of the drug. This quickly took me back to reality, but it did not bring me back so far that it would be difficult for me to return on my own. I, on the other hand, made use of this occasion to inform Brad about what was going on. When I finally got the chance to talk about the experience with someone, I could not contain my excitement and could not wait till it ended. I was encouraged by the woman to return, and she said that I should refrain from sharing my experience with other people at this moment. Because she wanted me to have a whole experience of what she intended to impart to me, she was encouraging me to slow down my thoughts. The message that she sent to me was that I should learn how to calm my thoughts, and it did not appear that I would be receiving any further instruction from her. As I continued to enter and exit the trip, I also continued to talk to Brad about my experience every time I did so. Her wrath stemmed from the fact that she had expressly instructed me not to disclose anything at this time and that she only desired for me to calm my thoughts. At this point in my life, I was not prepared to receive this message; but, I was completely prepared to receive it. My hubris and my attempt to exert control over the experience caused the entities to express their displeasure, and they bid me farewell on that note.

- **Trip Report #3: DMT Entities**

It dawned on me all of a sudden that I was participating in Terence McKenna's trip. It would be a shame if he didn't have a spot-on understanding of these wacky elves. As soon as I had this knowledge, the elves could not contain their amusement and came out laughing. While they were rolling over the ceiling and holding their tummies, they were laughing themselves crazy, giggling, and rolling about. Having said that, there was another thing. I had the impression that there was more to this location than simply the elves, and time was about to run out. I ventured farther into the domain of DMT, going beyond the realm of Elvin Mischief.

- **Trip Report #4: DMT Entities**

My perception of the 'elves' was different this time; I saw them as multidimensional entities that were created by strands of visible language; they were more creaturely than I had ever seen them before. It was the first time I had spotted them. The message, which had previously been described as "OK, OK, safe, safe...", was undergoing modifications at the time.

When the word "changing" is used, it provides the idea that this was a process that sequentially took place. For my part, I do not believe that this is the situation. While I was in the trance, I had the impression that the full message, together with all of its alterations, was there at the same moment, right from the start. Under the influence of DMT, time takes on a different meaning, and the idea of linear chronological sequence, which is something that we generally perceive to be true, is neither legitimate nor practical. This is because the sense of time is altered while one is under the influence of DMT. Our linear patterns of attention and the fact that we do not yet know how to see, hear, or perceive several messages concurrently and deliberately are the things that gave rise to the concept of linearity. As a consequence of this, we string them out for convenience in terms of perception. In every instance, every piece of information is readily accessible.

I did not see any faces in the conventional sense, but the elves were moving in and out of the multidimensional visual language matrix, "waving" their "arms" and "limbs/hands/fingers?" and "smiling" or "laughing," even though I did not see any faces. It seemed as though the elves were 'telling' me (or I was understanding them to suggest) that I had seen them in the past, most likely when I was a little child. Suddenly, my recollections of encountering the elves came flooding back to me: they appeared to be the same as they do now: they were constantly changing, folding, multidimensional, multicolored (what colors!), always laughing, weaving or waving, demonstrating things to me, demonstrating the visible language that they are created or creatures of, and teaching me how to speak and read.

CONCLUSION

When it comes to psychedelics, one of the most intriguing aspects is the widespread presence of DMT elves. Why is it that so many individuals who take DMT have experiences with beings?

Furthermore, why are there so many parallels between these claims from different sources?

Although they may have varied outward appearances, the majority of persons who have had experiences with these beings describe feeling the same way.

The beings in question are not only extraordinarily clever but also kind, inquisitive, and fun. The psychedelic explorer is frequently

66

provided with information that has a direct and beneficial influence on the individual's attitude toward life after the experience has been completed.

At this point, there is no way to determine whether or not these beings are genuine. They may be a fictitious result of psychedelic drugs; but, it is also possible that they are actual living things that exist in a realm that we are unable to interact with inside our regular waking awareness.

The message that these beings are trying to convey to you and how it may be utilized to improve your life or the lives of those around you is the most essential thing. It is not crucial what you choose to believe about these things.